The Day
Kadi
Lost Part of Her Life

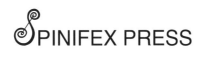
SPINIFEX PRESS

Editorial Direction
Leopoldo Blume

Photographs
Kim Manresa

Text
Isabel Ramos Rioja

Design
Natàlia Arranz

Translation
Nikki Anderson

Production Coordination
Cristina Rodríguez Fischer

Photoart
Scan 4, Barcelona

Printing
Grafos, S.A. Arte sobre papel, Barcelona

First published in Spanish by Blume, Barcelona, 1998

English language edition by Spinifex Press, Melbourne, 1998
PO Box 212 – North Melbourne – VIC 3051 – AUSTRALIA
Tel. +61-3-9329 6088 – Fax +61-3-9329 9238
women@spinifexpress.com.au
www.spinifexpress.com.au/~women

National Library of Australia
Cataloguing-in-Publication data:

Manresa. Kim
[El día que Kadi perdió parte de su vida. English]
The Day Kadi Lost Part of Her Life

ISBN: 1-875559-74-4

1. Female circumcision - Spain. 2. Infibulation - Spain.
3. Clitoridectomy - Spain. 4. Sex customs - Spain. I. Ramos Rioja.
Isabel. II. Anderson. Nikki. III. Title. IV. Title: El día que Kadi
perdió parte de su vida. English.

392.10946

The photographs on pages 29 and 40 are of a
circumcision practised on a one-year-old in the
same country.

The Day Kadi Lost Part of Her Life

photos **Kim Manresa**

prologue **Olayinka Koso-Thomas**

text **Isabel Ramos Rioja**

collaboration **David Serra**

SPINIFEX PRESS

Prologue

Dr Olayinka Koso-Thomas

*Recipient of the Príncipe de Asturias de Cooperación
Award, 1998 (Spain)*

The sacrifice of genital mutilation which Kadi experienced so early in her tender life has been going on in many parts of Africa for decades, even before the advent of Christianity or Islam. The practice of female genital mutilation (FGM) is a traditional one, endemic and culturally linked to many communities in Africa. This practice is detrimental to the health of women and the girl-child, who accept it without challenging the authority and tenets of its origin. The female population in areas where this practice is endemic have jealously guarded its secrets and are prepared to kill those women who are trying to highlight health hazards which prevent active participation in the development of family, community, country.

Kadi's story is typical of every little girl who lives in a community where to be loved, married, and held in high esteem requires you to be genitally mutilated. Failure to undergo the operation leads to harassment, ridicule, abuse, trauma, and eventual ostracism from one's community.

The attitude of the circumciser *(buankisa)* is typical of women who strongly believe they are doing Kadi a big favour by making her a marriageable commodity. The only role for African girls in that setting is matrimony with the eventual reproduction of children, which becomes an asset to her and the community. No man in that community is allowed to marry a girl who has not been genitally mutilated. FGM is the core prerequisite to matrimony, status, acceptability and peace of mind despite the fact that one's human rights have been violated and abused.

The fact that FGM, once performed, is permanent and makes the woman disengage from herself sexually, depressed psychologically, impotent and frustrated, makes no difference to the perpetrators of this wicked act, who strongly believe that they are acting in the best interest of the female child. The fact that many young girls die as a result of this practice makes no difference to their attitudes. Those who die are termed as wicked witches whom the community are glad to be rid of, hence the killing of chickens as sacrifice to appease the ancestral gods. The health of the girl is not taken into consideration, and she may be suffering from malnutrition, bacterial infection, or sickle cell anaemia and the circumciser is only interested in getting paid for work done, to maintain her status in the community.

In many African countries the practice of FGM is a political concern, and politicians seeking their own interest do not address this issue as it may cost them votes and the loss of parliamentary seats. As a result they turn a blind eye to the activities of the circumcisers *(buankisas)* who boast that nobody can stop them and that they will continue the mutilations, even in private.

I believe that with constant information, education, communication and sensitisation programmes, and with the collaboration and cooperation of African governments, the prevalence and incidence of the practice will be drastically reduced. The African girl-child may be free from mutilation and child abuse sometime in the 21st century.

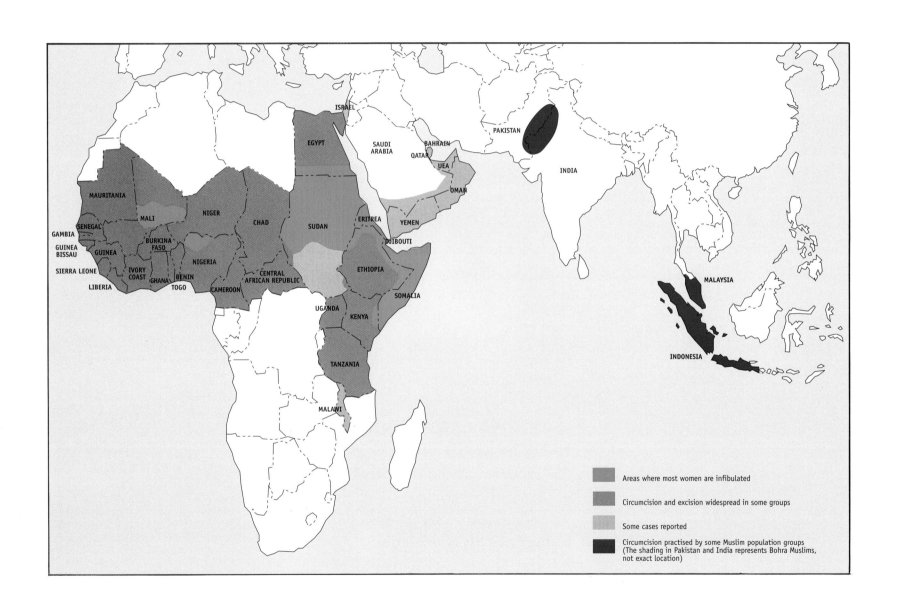

ISRAEL

EGYPT

SAUDI
ARABIA

QATAR BAHRAIN

PAKISTAN

INDIA

MAURITANIA

MALI

NIGER

UEA

OMAN

GAMBIA

SENEGAL

CHAD

SUDAN

ERITREA

YEMEN

GUINEA
BISSAU

BURKINA
FASO

DJIBOUTI

GUINEA

NIGERIA

SIERRA LEONE

IVORY
COAST

CENTRAL
AFRICAN REPUBLIC

ETHIOPIA

LIBERIA

GHANA BENIN

TOGO

CAMEROON

MALAYSIA

SOMALIA

UGANDA

KENYA

TANZANIA

INDONESIA

MALAWI

Areas where most women are infibulated

Circumcision and excision widespread in some groups

Some cases reported

Circumcision practised by some Muslim population groups
(The shading in Pakistan and India represents Bohra Muslims,
not exact location)

What is
female genital
mutilation?

Around one hundred and thirty million girls and women have suffered mutilation of the clitoris. Two million girls suffer this practised annually. Its origins do not lie in Islam and it is not necessarily a rite of initiation; nor is it always used to control women's virginity, although almost certainly her sexuality. It is a little of all these things and practised in around thirty countries of the world. In each area it is done in a different way and has different explanations.

The most moderate (if one may consider it as such) excision is that of Muslim tradition known as 'sunna', which entails the partial or total excision of the body of the clitoris. It is practised in some areas of the Middle East and the expansion of Islam has introduced it to certain communities in Pakistan, Indonesia and Malaysia. The type most practised in countries of central Africa, it is associated with cleanliness. With the act, girls are integrated into the community and are transformed into women ready for matrimony. A woman who has not been mutilated risks being rejected by her husband-to-be, and even her friends. Infibulation, the most severe type, consists of the removal of the clitoris, plus the excision of part or the entire labia majora. The raw edges of the vulva are sewn together and a small opening is left to allow a passage for urine and menstrual blood. This is called pharonic circumcision, and is widely practised in Egypt, Somalia, Eritrea and Sudan. Following circumcision, women must, in some cases, be literally ripped open to allow penetration.

Clitoridectomy seems to have been practised even before written records exist. The belief was formed in Egypt that the foreskin was the feminine part of the male and the clitoris the masculine part of woman. Thus, removal avoided any type of sexual ambiguity.

Chronicle of a Sacrifice

text: Isabel Ramos Rioja

photos: Kim Manresa

Kadi's first scream went through me like a dagger. The subsequent cries formed like a knot in my stomach. I lacked air to breathe and my vision clouded. Kadi, the cheerful four-year-old who hadn't stopped playing with us 'whites' since the day we'd arrived, had just discovered pain, the horror of tradition. They had circumcised her; on a raffia mat, held down by an elderly woman of the village, using a splash of iodine for sterilisation. In line after her were two other little girls- two sisters of one and four years of age.

In the chronicles of the Rwanda massacres, it was said that it seemed as if African children didn't know how to cry. Kadi's cries went from weeping to barely a whimper; the *buankisa*, the name given to women who act as circumcisers in this sub-Saharan country, didn't give it a thought. Like any other of the many vultures flying around, the old woman even took some of the sweets which had been brought for Kadi.

For the adolescents busying themselves with farming and domestic tasks at the house where the circumcision was to take place, it was a day just like any other. One of them took care of the smallest girl and put her on her back immediately after her wound, caused by the repeated cuts of the old razor blade, had been covered with a dirty rag. The men, relaxing on mats in the shade of storm clouds, chatted as if nothing had happened. They didn't understand my look of despair, that of the white woman who attended the operation, and with a joking smile asked, "How did you think it would be?".

Kadi, with her 'ekai' hairstyle, hair held stiff and upright, had to travel hundreds of kilometres to be subjected to this ancestral ritual. In her region there is strict control by the Ministry of Health, so that she had to be sent to relatives who acted as go-between with the father of another girl to be circumcised. Once the pact was made, we all set off on the journey to the village where the clitoridectomy was to take place.

Kadi, on my lap, shared the back seat with the old woman who was about to deprive her of part of her life, and another beautiful young woman, Meriem, who had been mutilated by the same *buankisa*. "Do I hate this woman? No, the first time I saw her after the operation I was scared and ran away, but that has passed... although I'll never forget that day," Meriem tells. The *buankisa*, for her part, didn't pay the slightest attention to little Kadi, not even to try and gain her confidence to make the job easier.

Kadi played and played around the village huts. Rising at daybreak and travelling for four hours with stops only to buy dried fish, rice and red sorghum for the 'host' family hadn't dented her enthusiasm. She ate peanuts and used the shells as ammunition against the photographer and myself, then drank the chilled water packaged in the local style- in little plastic bags which you pricked a hole in and sucked the water from one end.

The villagers – where the circumcision was to take place - lived amongst fields of red sorghum, beans, and cotton. One family occupied a group of four or five huts, each one with its

purpose: for cooking, to house supplies, another for hanging clothes – tied to palm leaves from the roof – another for sleeping – on straw mats thrown over stones – and another for eating, or, in this case for the girls to lie down in after the operation.

Kadi played in this environment, completely unaware of what was about to happen and continued running around until the *buankisa* told her sternly to undress in a corner near one of the huts. Ochre-coloured stains – from dried blood – on the walls of the adobe surrounding the huts signalled the site where the family performed animal sacrifices.

It was there too that the circumcisions were held. First they grabbed Kadi. An old woman sat behind her. She pinned Kadi's arms with her hands and placed her legs over hers to prevent her from moving. The first incision did not complete the circumcision and cuts were repeated until all of the clitoris and the labia minora were removed. Then they let her go, left her on the ground and turned to the other girls. The father of these girls

was Islamic, like Kadi, and justified his decision to have his daughters circumcised: "It's always been done. You have to do it," he said as he took the youngest in his arms affectionately.

Neither Christianity nor Islam has managed to end the traditional faith in witchdoctors. This man, separated from his wife, consulted a witchdoctor of his community some time ago about having both daughters circumcised at the same time. The witchdoctor advised against it: "Just the older one." (the three-year-old). The father should have consulted once more, despite the witchdoctor's suggestions nothing was going to give the one-year-old any such luck. In order that the situation is favourable, a chicken had to first be sacrificed. With the words 'bismil·lah' (in the name of God, in Arabic) the father gave them to the man considered the holiest – in this case Iliase, the bus driver – for him to kill according to Muslim tradition.

Three chickens and the equivalent of three cents were given to the *buankisa* for the operations. The money is symbolic. Of greatest importance are the chickens and that the expenses for the *buankisa's* pilgrimage around the country are paid for. Since the government initiated one of the most significant anti-female circumcision campaigns in any African country, she travels with her raffia bag, knife and jar of iodine to wherever her services are required, as the local *buankisas* are now well controlled.

"Even if I have to do it hidden in a room, I'll continue," she assures me. "I'm the sixth generation of my family to do this. I began with my own daughter. Charity begins with oneself, doesn't it?" she asks me with a smile, which nobody questions. Kumba is seventy years old and knows that women like herself enjoy enormous prestige.

For four years the government has run an informative and persecutory campaign against this practice to which nearly all women and girls of certain regions have been subjected. Christians, Muslims and animists. So far nobody has been freed. However, things are beginning to change in this country where twenty per cent of the population is Muslim. In the weekly sermons held in the tiny and numerous mosques, the Imams are taking it on themselves to re-educate their followers: female genital mutilation is neither of Islamic origin nor obligatory. Iliase's little girl is lucky to have a father who attends mosque each Friday and follows the Imam's words. "I won't do it to my little girl," he confesses to me with a clear conscience.

Meriem, the young Muslim woman who accompanied Kadi and passed through Kumba's hands some twenty years ago, won't have her daughter circumcised. Penetration with her partner is difficult because of circumcision. "Men prefer women who haven't been circumcised," she says without wanting to enter into details. Her partner, a Christian, is one of the generation who was sent abroad to study. There, he experienced the type of sexual relations which are impossible to recreate on his return. When he meets a woman he adores, she is sexually detached.

Kadi finds herself amongst strangers once more, with the family of the girls who shared the circumcision. Their father will return after a week to see how things have gone. If there are no complications, he will take Kadi back to her family, transformed into a proper member of the community.

Day is breaking and Kadi's still asleep on her straw mat. She gets up early, like the adults, thinking that today is just a day like any other. She puts on a t-shirt and is ready to go out into the courtyard.

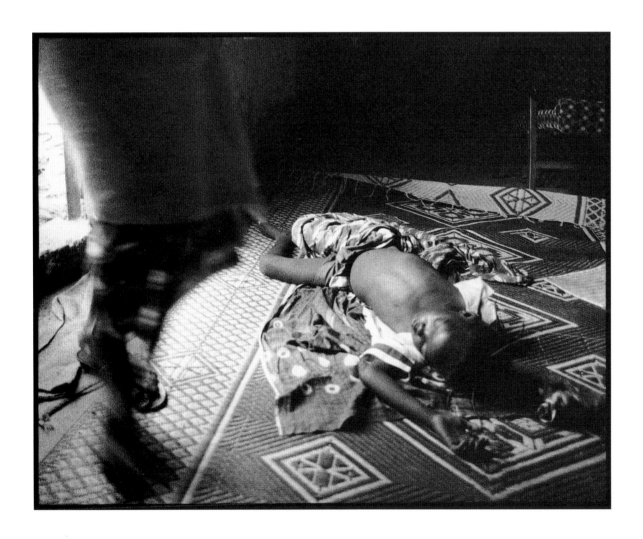

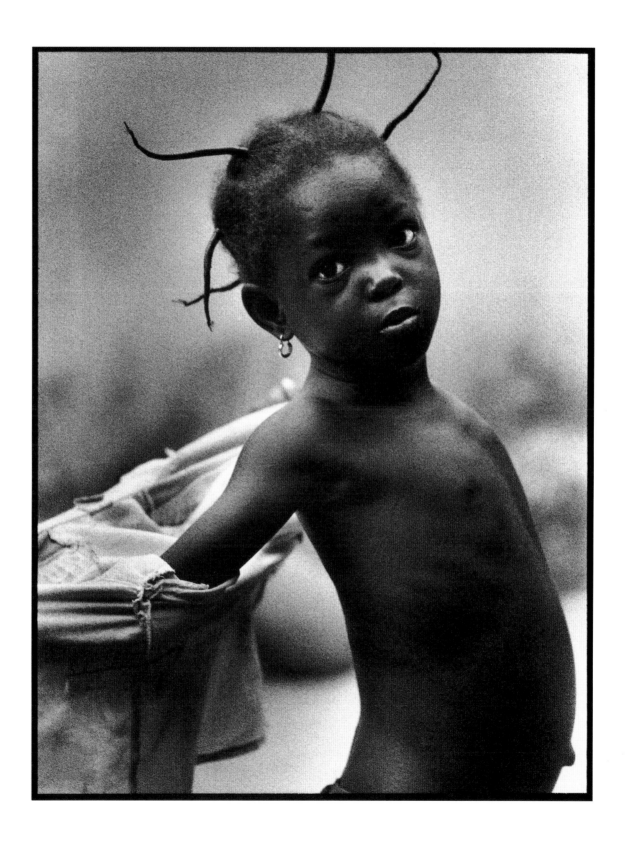

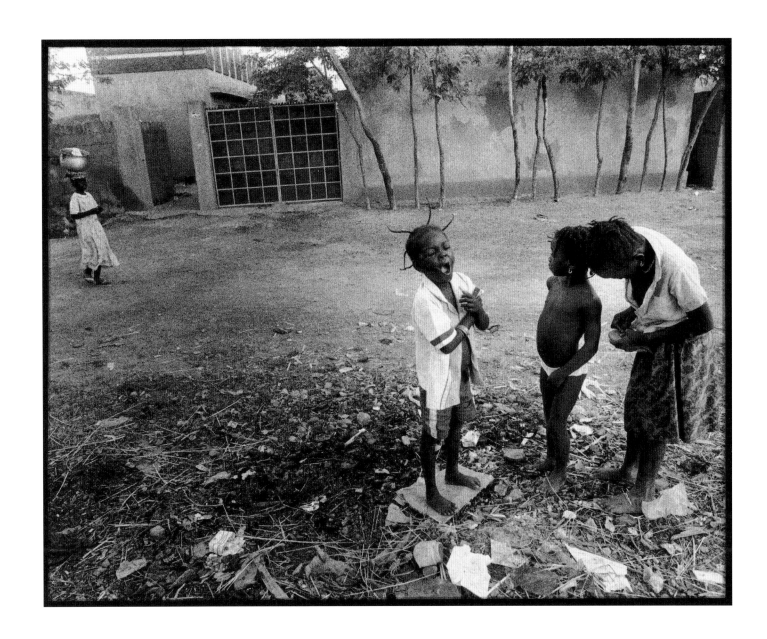

The courtyard's too small for Kadi, and while
she stretches and wakes up, she ventures
out onto the dirt streets with the other girls
of the neighbourhood. The city is waking up
and it is the women who are first seen,
carrying things from here to there.

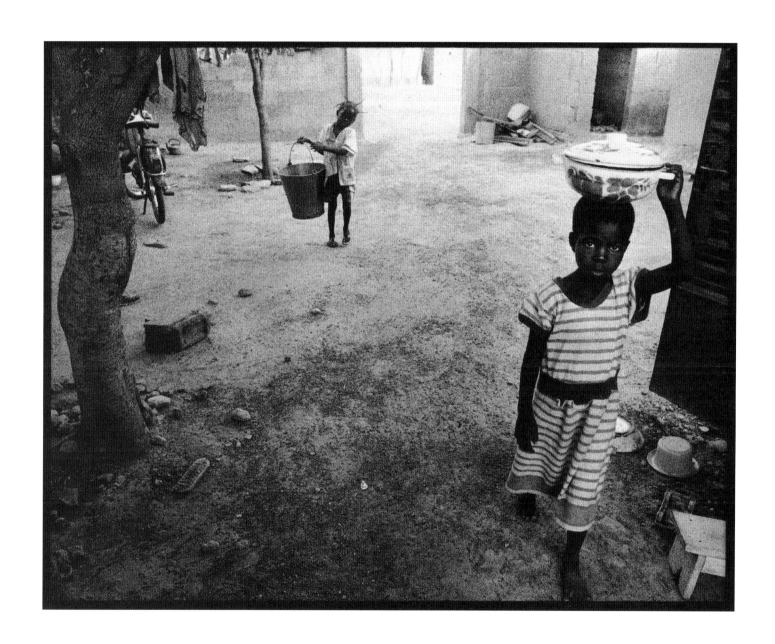

For Abugumá the day begins at first
light. She has to take care of her
younger siblings and can't even stop to
help Kadi with the big pot.

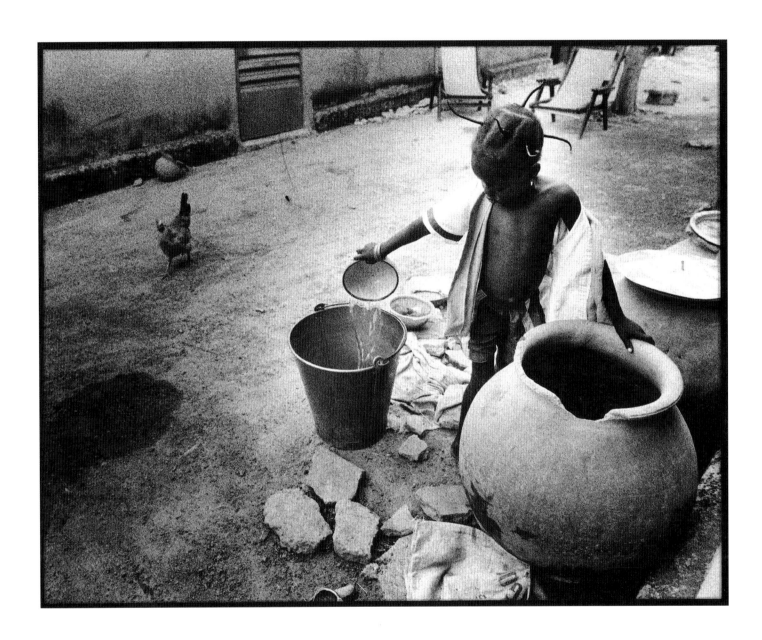

Kadi uses half a dried pumpkin to scoop
water from the clay pot to wash herself
while the hens run around the entrance
to the home.

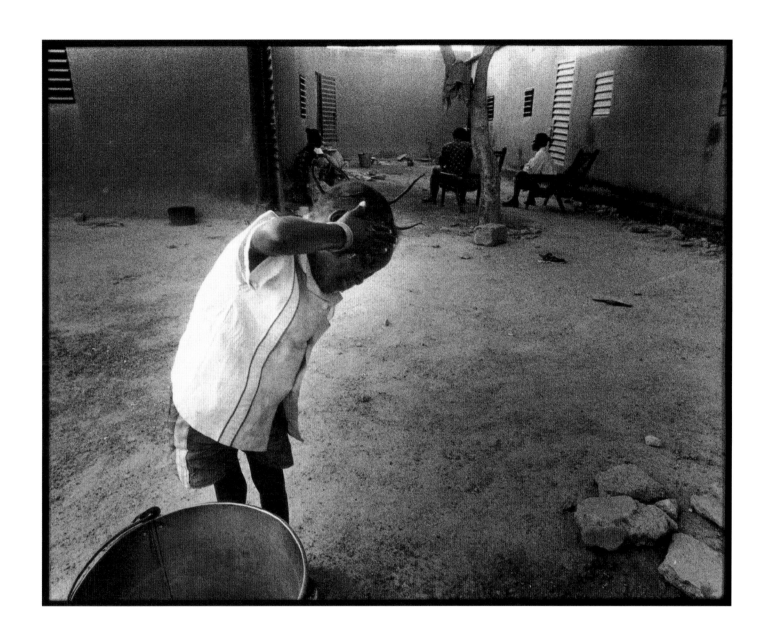

The men of the neighbourhood start the
day with one of their favourite pastimes -
sitting down for a quiet chat. The
children, like Kadi, stay on the sidelines.

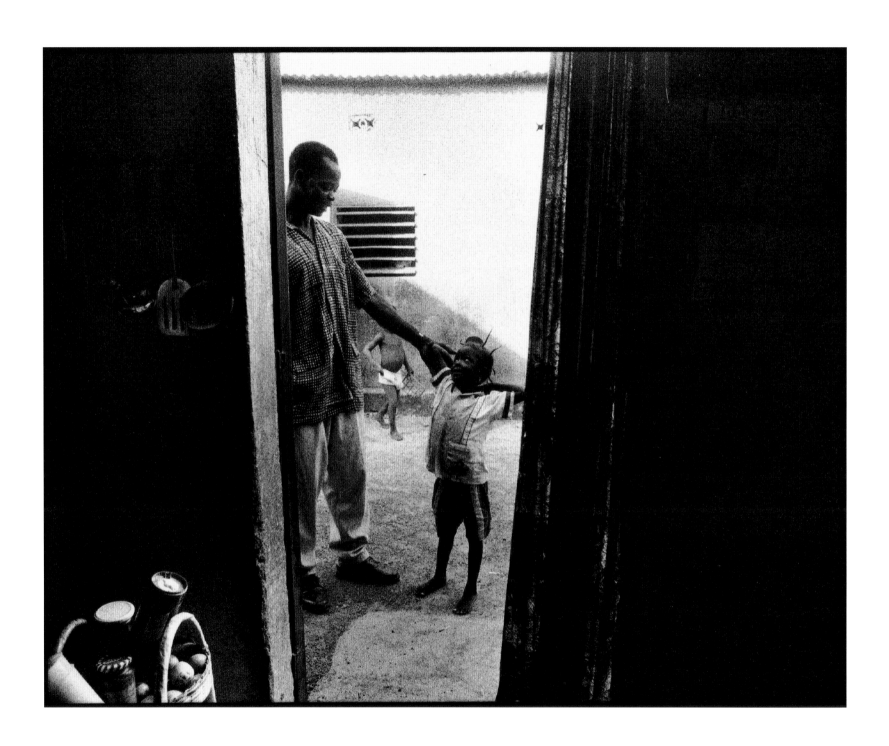

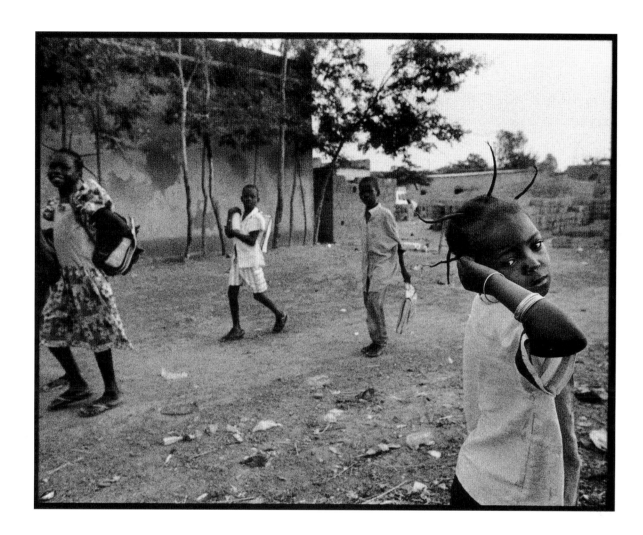

The young man shows affection to the
little girl. Kadi doesn't know he is the
father of the two girls who will be
subjected to circumcision along with
herself in the distant village.

The most privileged children, nineteen
per cent of this sub-Saharan country,
attend school. Kadi has to stay home as
today is the day she will confront the
horror of tradition.

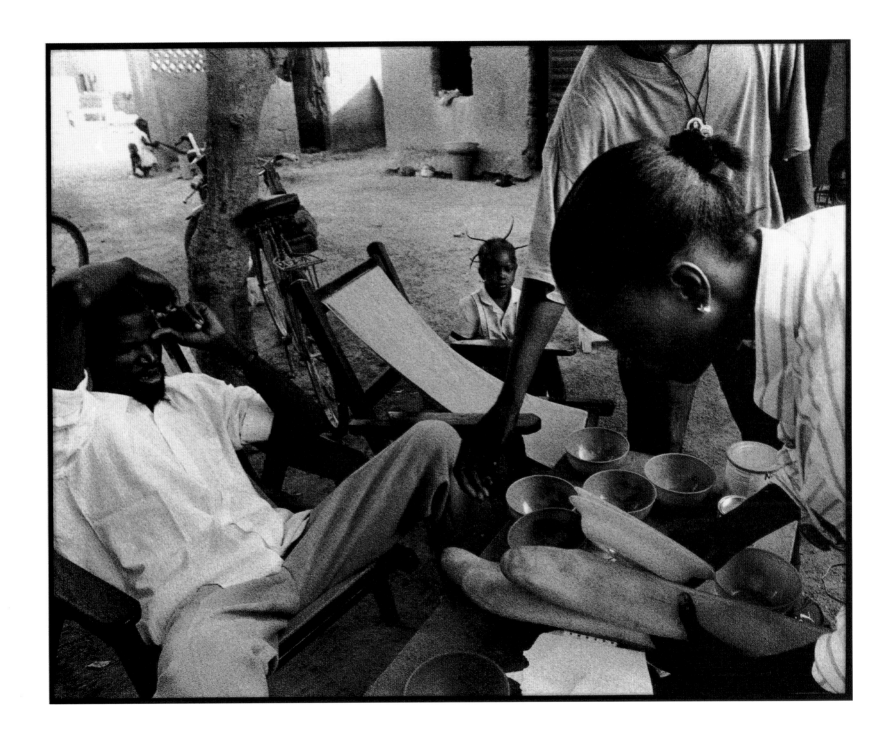

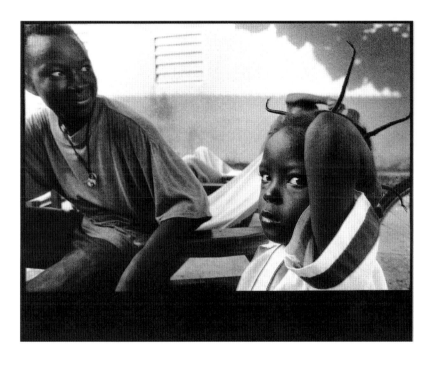

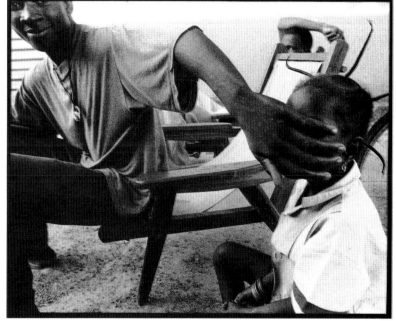

Before embarking on the long trip to the village where the ritual will take place, Iliase, the bus driver shares his breakfast with everyone.

Kadi, with her 'ekai' hairstyle is serious for the camera, but her bright character raises Hervé's affection.

After four hours of travelling, she's thirsty and empties the bag of cool water bought on the way. The *buankisa*, the woman who will perform the circumcision, takes a break before beginning her 'work'.

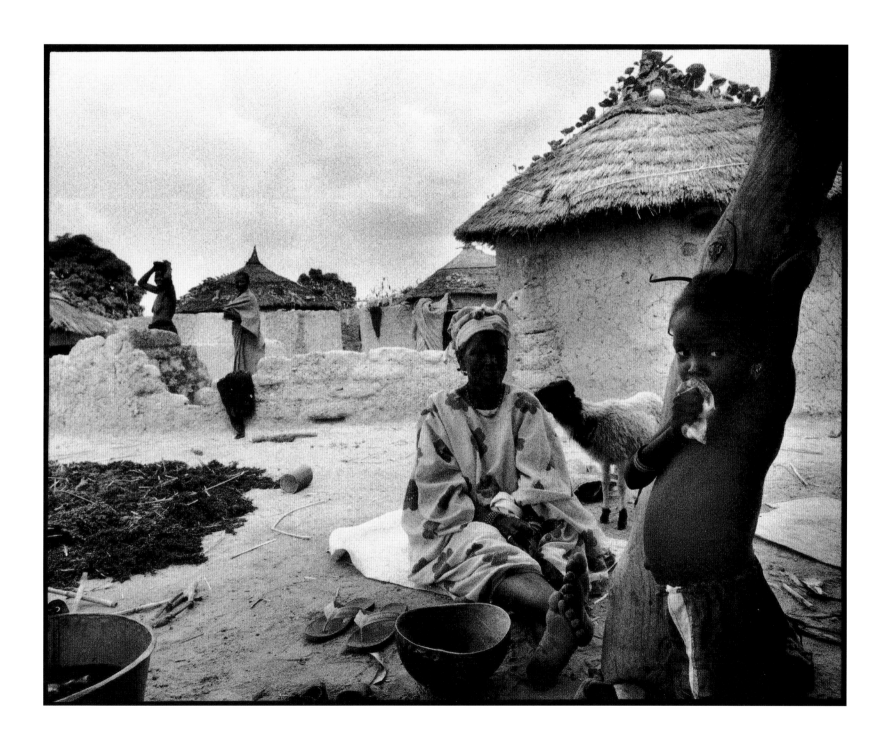

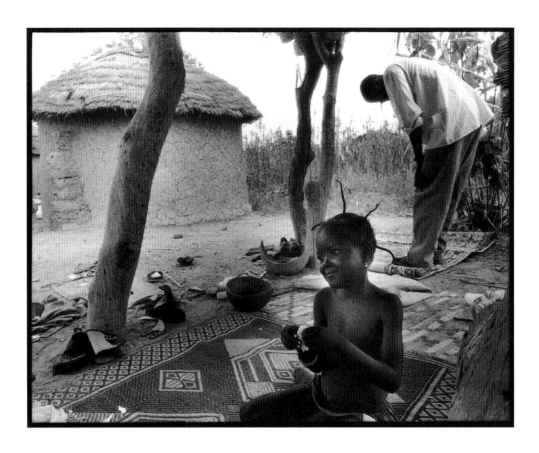

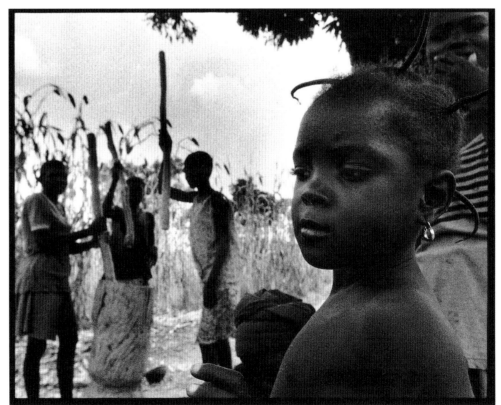

Iliase, the bus driver, doesn't forget his obligations to Islam. After performing the mandatory ablutions he prays on a mat which separates him from the earth and brings him closer to God.

Between smiles, the adolescents of the village pound millet which is cultivated in the fields around the huts. Kadi won't eat today.

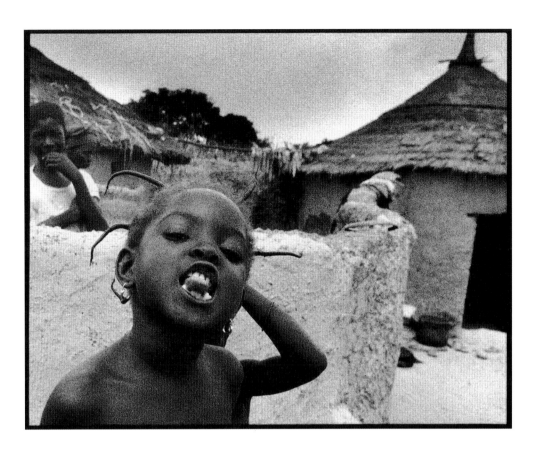

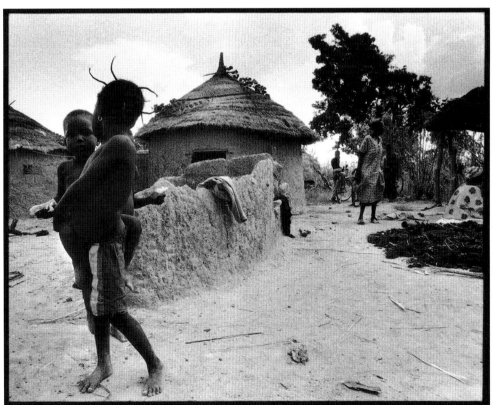

Kadi looks after the little one-year-old who will share her suffering. In the background are the two women who will be in charge of the sacrifice.

Mischievously she flirts with the camera and plays with the photographer. She is not shy with strangers and the presence of foreigners doesn't bother her.

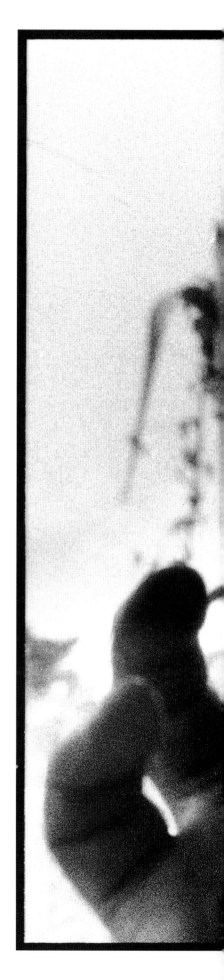

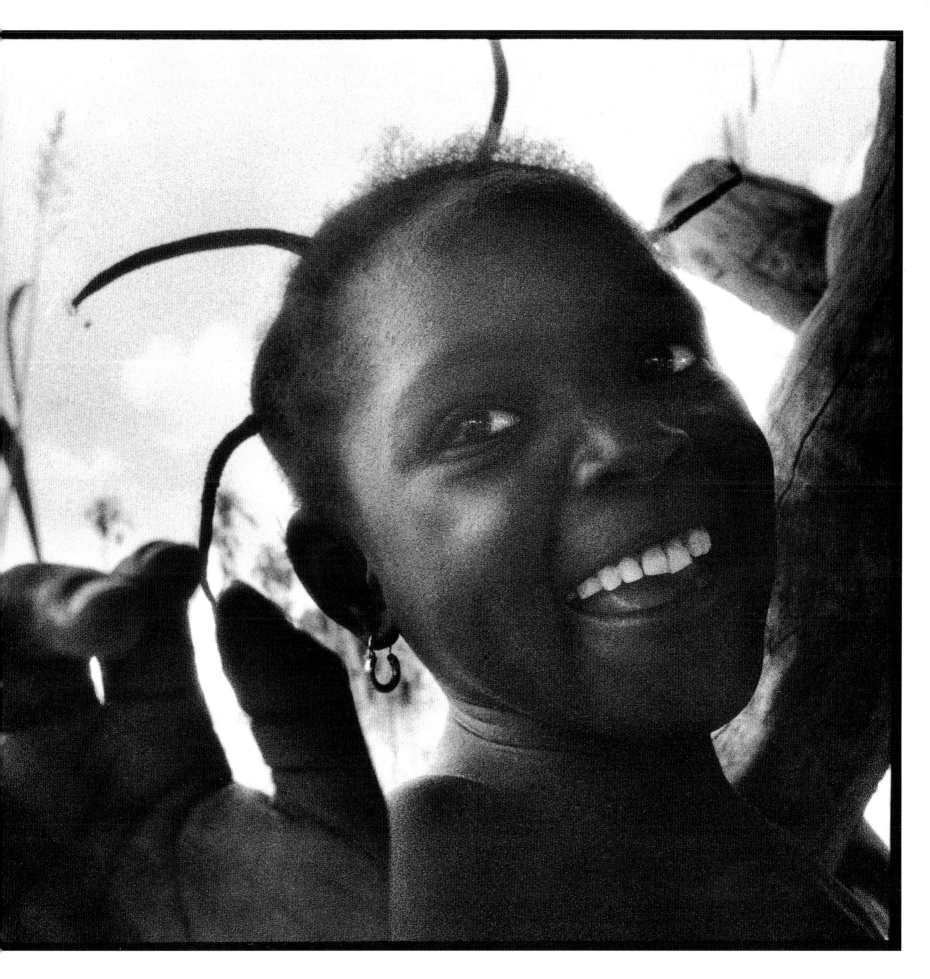

Ritual
of Sacrifice

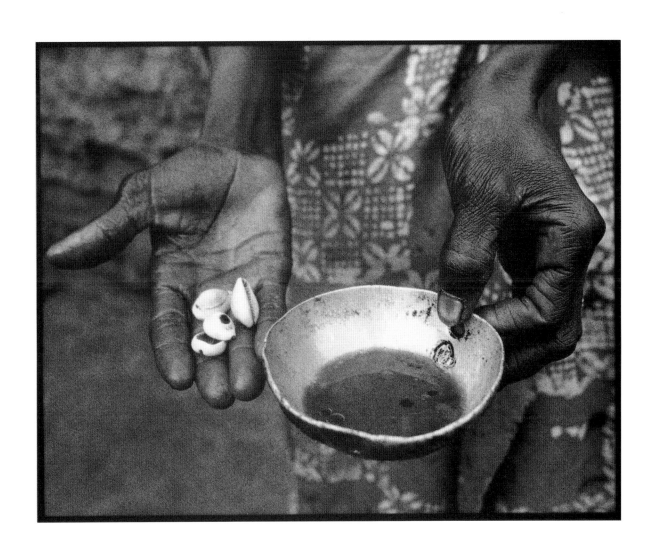

The *buankisa* uses a hoe to dig a hole
for the blood which will flow during
the circumcision, in which an old
woman will be present to hold down
the girls. The walls are already covered
in blood from another sacrifice – the
chickens.

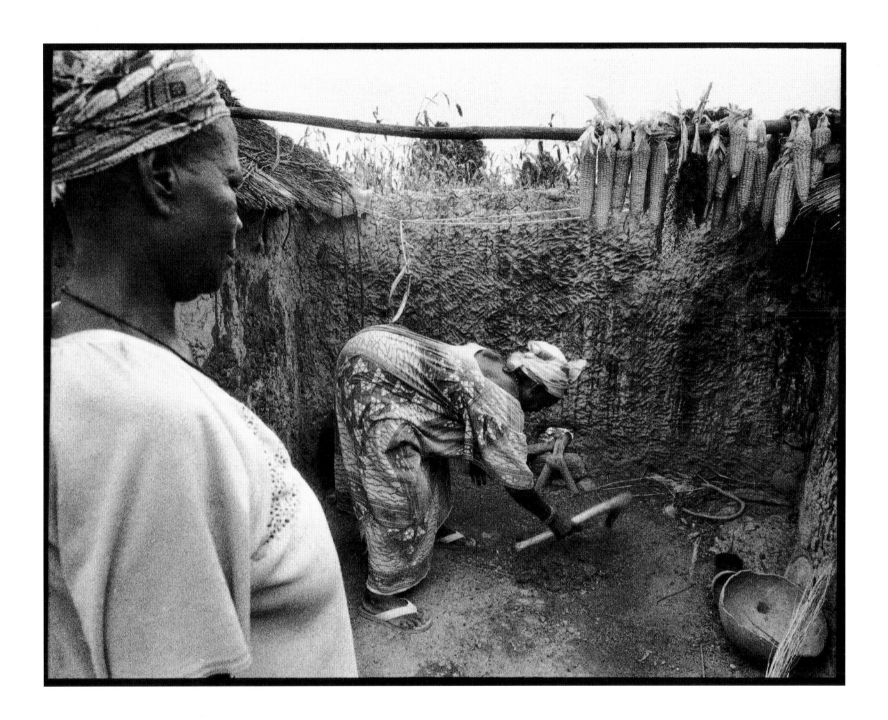

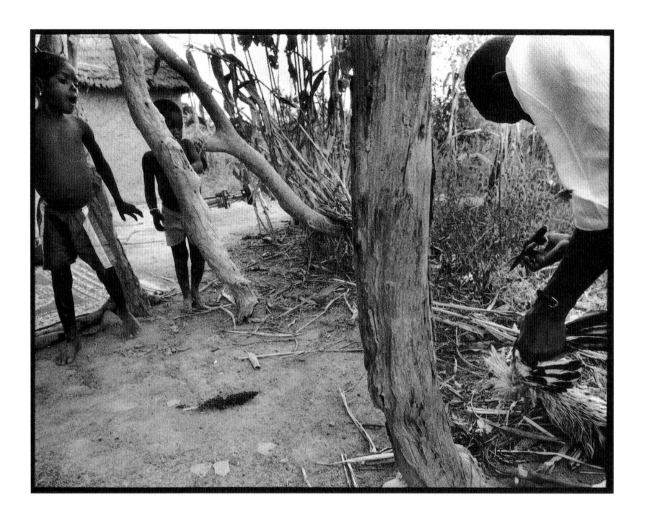

Iliase, as the holy one, has to sacrifice
a rooster in front of the girls according
to Muslim tradition.

Kadi participates in a ritual, a
precursor to her own, by holding down
the rooster for Iliase.

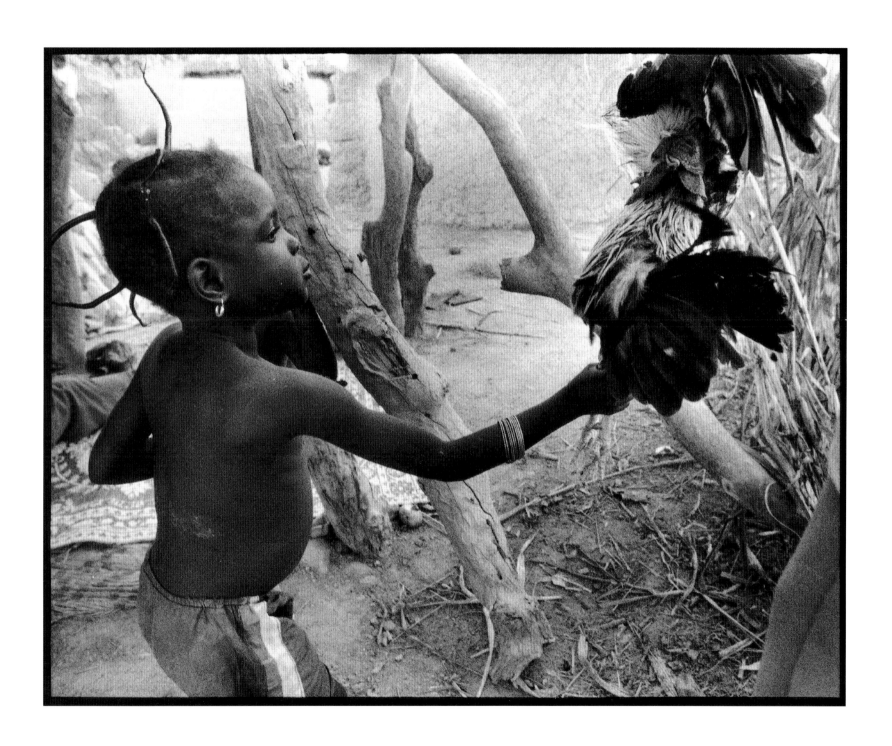

Now she has been stripped of her
clothes. Kadi is defenceless against the
respect for the older women and the
cruelty of the customs.
Realising herself naked in the corner,
Kadi begins to appear afraid.

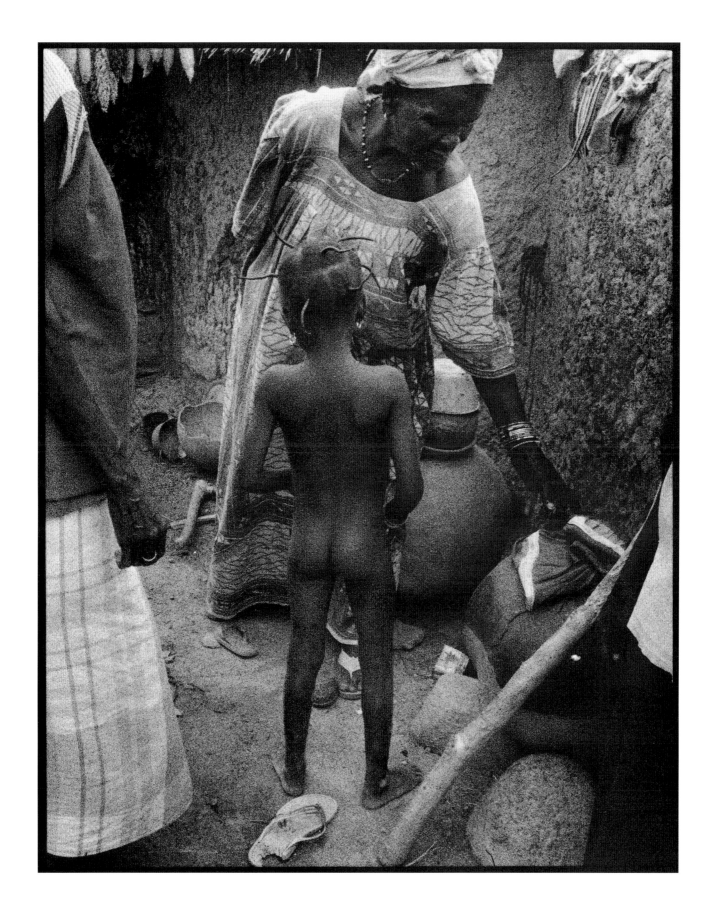

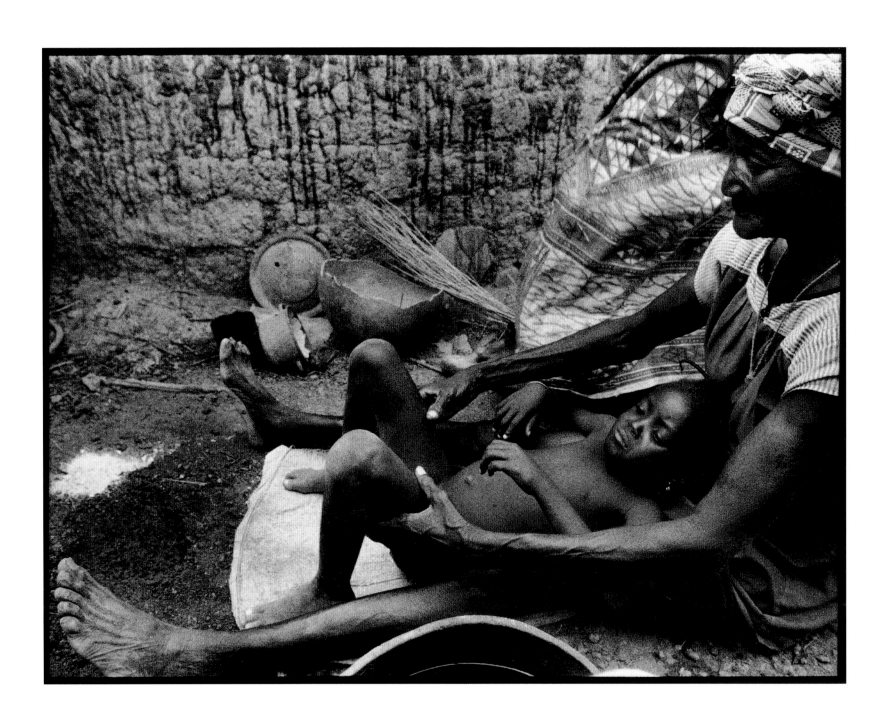

The old woman, undaunted, holds down the girl with mechanical movements, learned through much practice. Kadi's blood spills like that of the sacrificed animals and dries on the walls.

The *buankisa* holds the older woman's leg against the girl's lap. If she manages to immobilise her, the 'work' will be much simpler and the cut, cleaner.

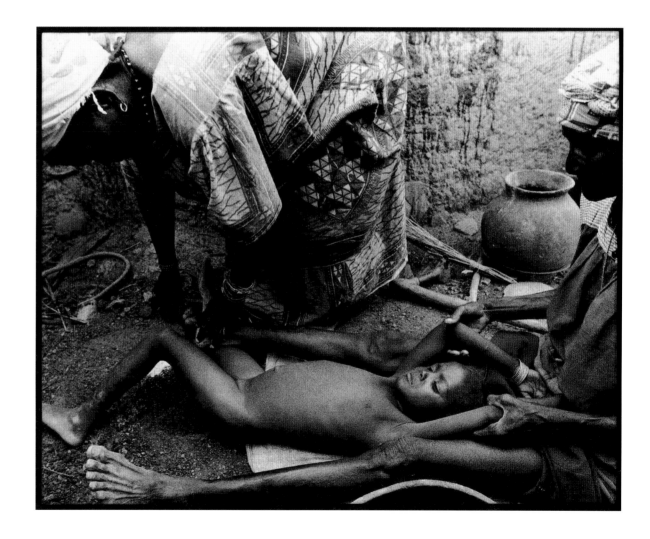

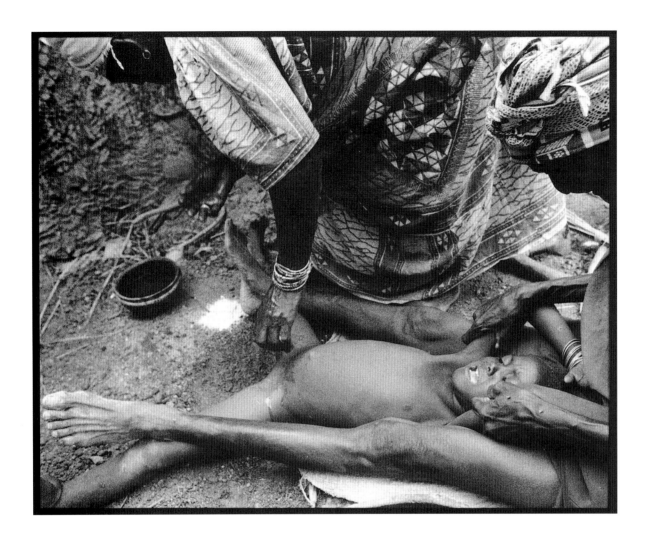

With the first incision, Kadi's screams cut the heavy air of the sky, threatening a storm. The *buankisa's* hands are covered with blood, again.

The pain is unbearable and Kadi fears the incisions will never end.

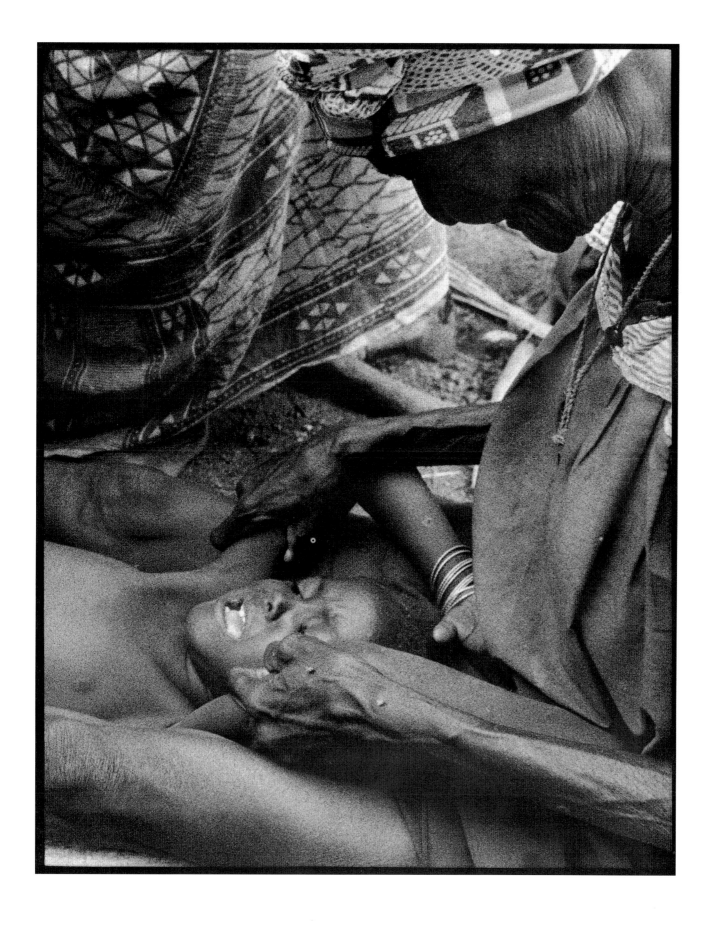

The strength of the old woman is insufficient against the instinctive reaction of Kadi's pain, and the cuts of the razor, used on each girl until the point of bluntness, are repeated despite her movement.

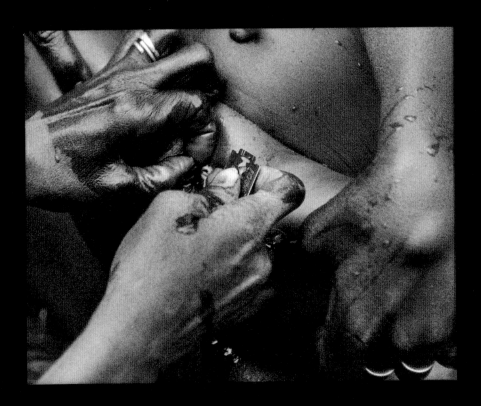

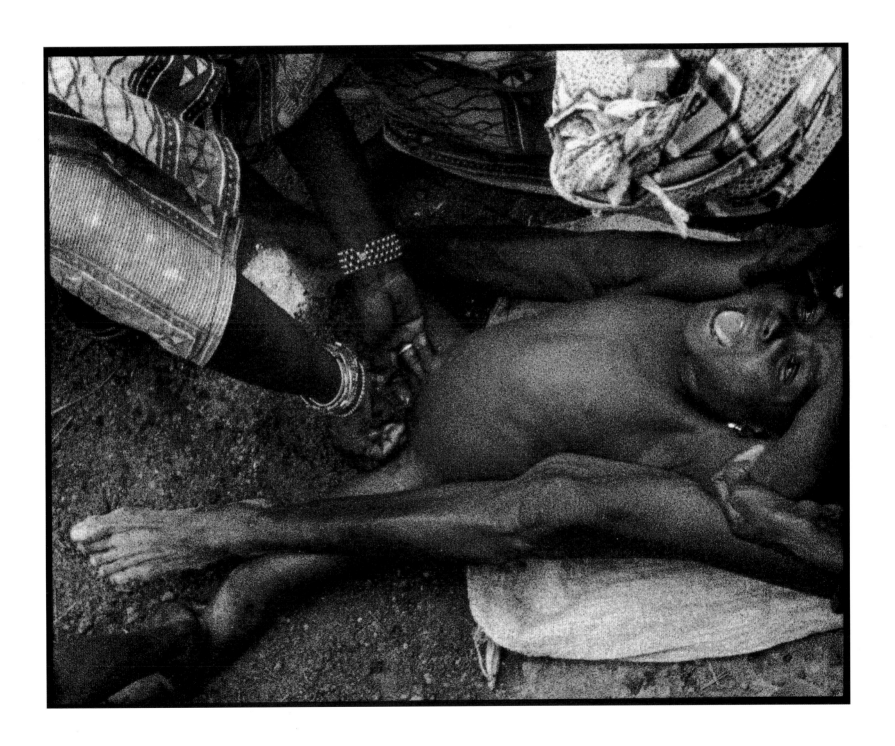

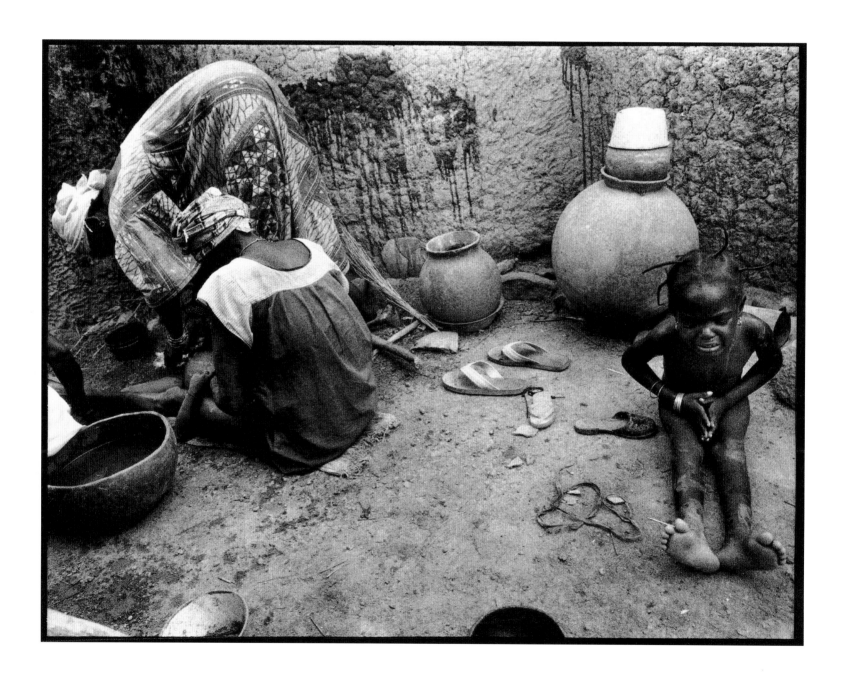

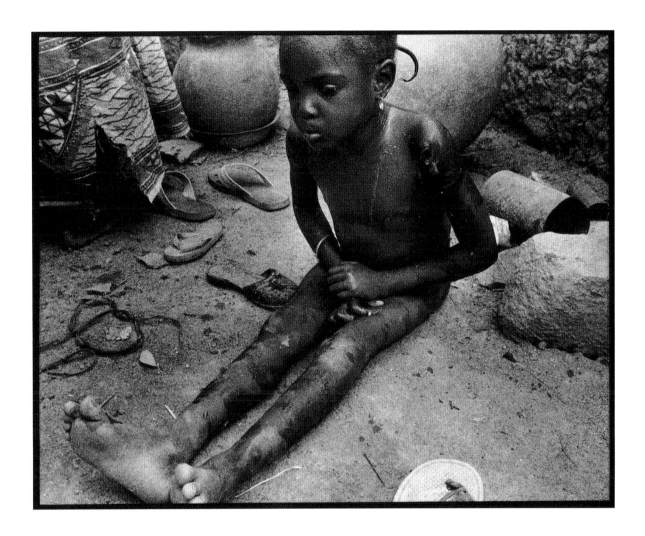

Kadi cries while she obediently
remains where the *buankisa* has left
her. The operation is repeated on the
three-year-old. Her one year old
sister follows.

Kadi's cries give way to sobbing,
then fade to a whimper despite the
blood stains all over the place.

The old woman indicates with pointed finger that the crying should stop, because she says so. Immediately. For the sake of tradition they have to put up with the pain.

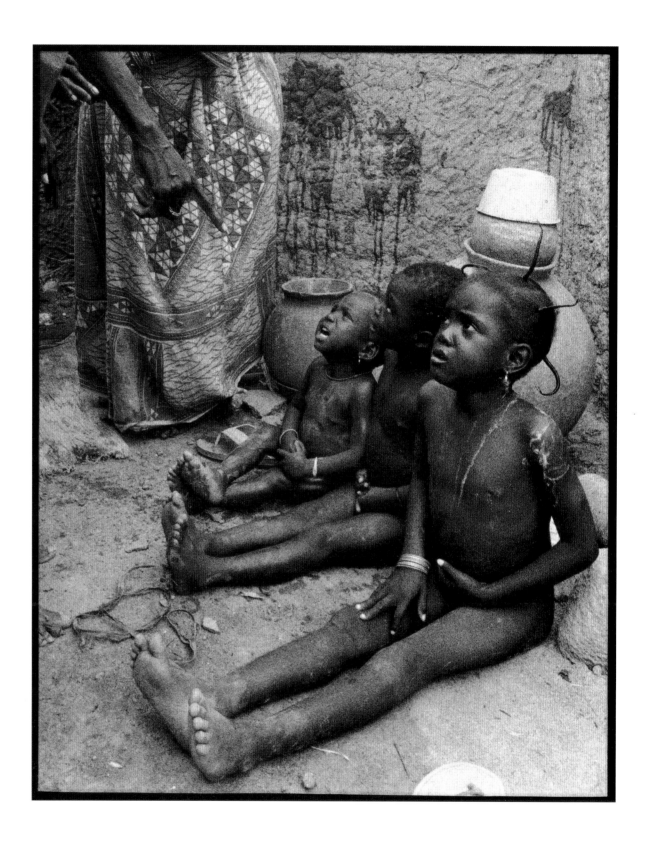

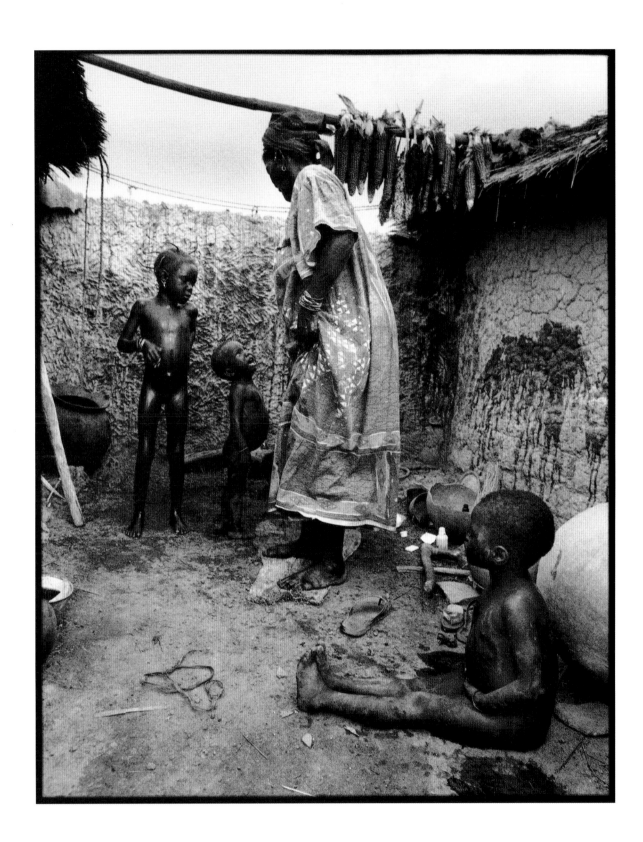

Kadi, with the other girls, returns to the place where part of her life has been taken, to be treated with a splash of iodine and water. For several days to come the earth will show signs of their mutilation.

Covered with a blanket and a dirty
rag between her legs in an attempt
to stop the haemorrhaging, Kadi is
sent to a hut where she must remain
immobile for a week to allow the
wound to heal itself.
She will never be the same again.
She has lost a part of her life.

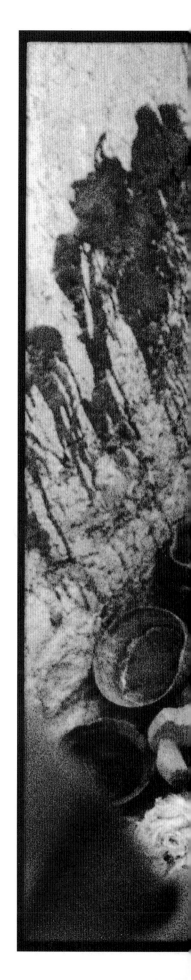

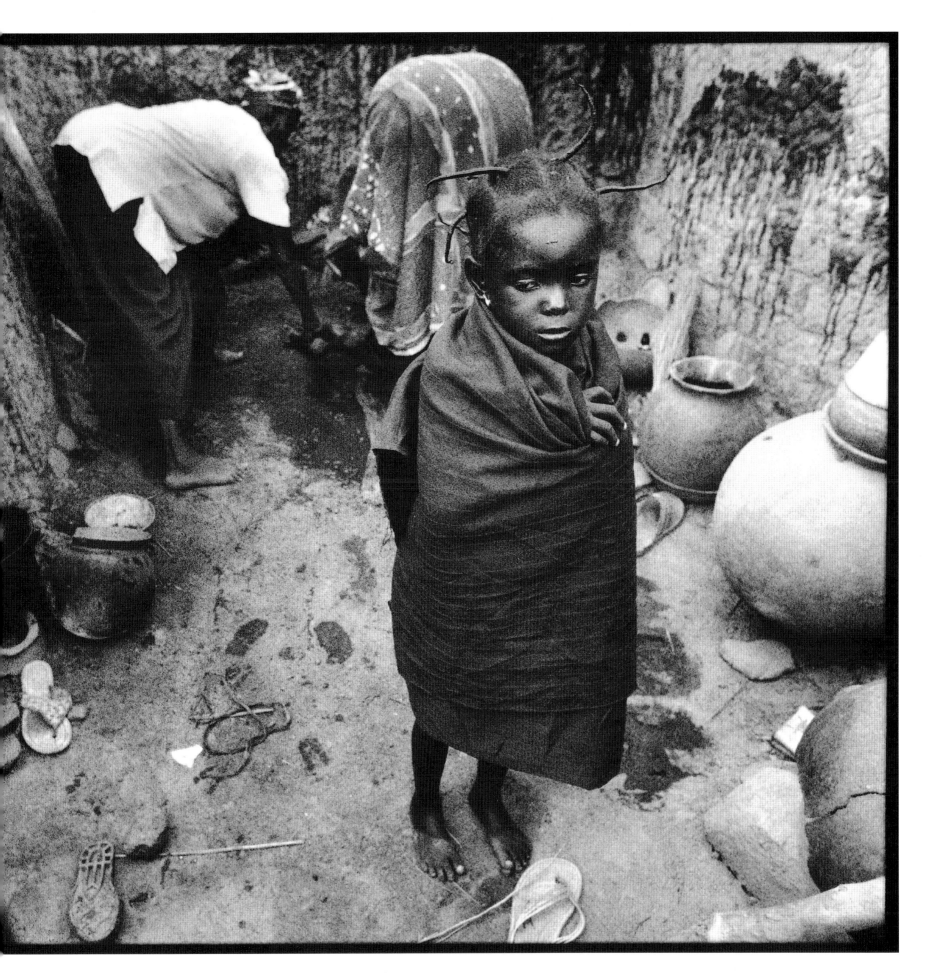

FORWARD

Foundation for Women´s Health, Research and Development

• FORWARD is a British non-governmental organisation which works internationally to aid in the eradication of the practice of female genital mutilation.

• FORWARD participated in a campaign, endorsed by the United Nations, which saw FGM recognised as a violation against human rights.

• In 1995, thanks to the campaign run by FORWARD, the British government passed a law which made the practice of clitoridectomy in British territory illegal.

• In 1992, FORWARD organised an international conference where member countries of the European Union signed a declaration against FGM.

What does FORWARD do?

• It sponsors sanitation and women's health programs run by African doctors in Africa with the main objective being the elimination of FGM.

• It offers psychologial, medical and economic aid to women who have been traumatised by FGM, in Africa and other continents.

• It collaborates with The World Health Organisation and the Ministries of Health in many countries to educate about FGM.

• Collaborates in research projects into the prevention of veseca-vaginal fistula in Africa.

• Funds the Africa Well Woman's Clinic at Northwick Park Hospital, Middlesex which attends to gynaecological needs of women who have suffered infibulation, and offers interpreters in various African languages for the women and medical team.

Donations to Foundation for Women's Health Research and Development (FORWARD) Donations Account can be made through the Strand branch (P.O. Box 414 - 38 Strand- London WC2N 5JQ) of the NatWest Bank, account number 31165745 (cod. 60-40-05)

For more information about FORWARD:
FORWARD
40 Eastbourne Terrace
London W2 3QR - England
Tel. + 44 171 725 2606
Fax. + 44 171 725 2796
E-mail: forward@dircon.co.uk